Light for Your Journey

A Christ-Filled Guide Through Cancer

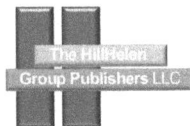

The HillRelori
Group Publishers LLC

Light for Your Journey

A Christ-Filled Guide Through Cancer

By Donne C. Smith

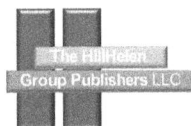

The HillHelen
Group Publishers LLC

Library of Congress Cataloging-in-Publication Data

ISBN: 979-8-9888614-2-3

Printed and bound in the United States of America by Ingram Lightning Source

First edition

Cover image: Tim Lewis, www.KingofMcAfee.com

Cover design: Jacque Hillman

Editing, layout, and design: Jacque Hillman and Katie Gould

The HillHelen Group LLC
470 North Parkway, Suite C
Jackson, TN 38305

The HillHelen Group LLC
635 North 65th Place
Mesa, AZ 85205

(731) 394-2894
www.hillhelengrouppublishers.com
hillhelengroup@gmail.com

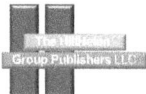

To my husband, who, through sickness and health, has walked by my side, respectfully and tenderly caring for me in all the roller-coasters our life together has produced!

To Diana for coming into our home and being my sister. She planned a meal train for six months of treatment, mopped my floors, made sure everyone had a ride, did the laundry, reprimanded the mouthy ones, and held my head both times I threw up. My family of origin adopted her!

To Brenda for sacrificially loving me and giving me a summer full of good memories and safety.

To my sisters Harriet, Patti, and Laura, and to Buz for coming at the right time for the right time to nurture us all. To Everett for keeping our parents on an even keel.

To Mary Jane for making me laugh while you dusted my living room.

To our church for being a part of the meal train and for extending the love of Christ to our family during a crisis. For flower beds, visits, and phone calls. It all helped to aid in endurance.

To all those who choose to work daily with people who are fighting for their lives in the face of their mortality. Dr. Reese, at the Jackson Clinic, was kind and thorough and always truthful. The nurses at the clinic worked together like a well-oiled machine, understanding what their counterparts needed with a nod or a look. And each one is able to give life-giving words into the ears of their patients. Elizabeth, Donna, Mindy, Jeanne, thank you.

To Jesus, the author and perfector of our faith, who promises to never leave us or forsake us, to be with us to the very end. How grateful I am that You walked with me through this and will walk with me to the end.

Table of Contents

Acknowledgments

Without the constant encouragement of my daughter, Stephanie Powell, and her editing prowess, this little book would not exist.

My power girls also deserve to be acknowledged for their part in encouraging me.

Again, my husband, Roger, who has given again to see this idea and dream come to pass.

BEFORE YOU BEGIN

I am the busy mother of four children: three adolescent daughters and one sweet surprise of a son. During the Christmas season of 2003, in the midst of holiday preparations, I discovered a small lump in my right breast. Because I had a "been there, done that before" attitude, I waited until after the holidays to get it checked out.

During my appointment with a surgeon friend, we decided to wait six weeks before excising the lump. During the second visit, he was willing to wait six more weeks. Thinking to save time and money, I said, "Let's just go ahead and biopsy it." I was convinced it was nothing more than fibrocystic tissue.

When the pathology report revealed abnormal cells, we scheduled a lumpectomy. I was still certain the lump would be harmless. After surgery, Dr. Jones came to tell me the report results. Direct and kind, he gently told me it was cancerous. Shock crystallized that moment forever in my memory. Suddenly, I had become a statistic. I stood at the threshold of a world I had only known as a spectator.

Like a tennis match in my head, I began to wonder if I had eaten better, if I had exercised more, if I had been more proactive in caring for my body . . . could I have prevented this from happening? Was this a genetic problem? Was it an environmental consequence? What did this to me? Why? How could I keep it from continuing? Every lob

I sent over the net was met with insufficient answers. The imaginary judge kept mumbling pronouncements that I could not hear.

After the first surgery to remove the tumor, I came home to a houseful of frightened faces. I held up fairly well but longed to be alone. Finally, I made my way to the bathtub. As I sat in the warm bubbles, the reality of my diagnosis began to crash in around me. Was this it? Was this all my life would consist of? Would I die? Would my children forget me? Would this destroy their trust in a loving and good God?

I had so much more I wanted to accomplish. My children needed me. I wanted to help them, to see them marry, to have grandchildren, to grow old with my sweet husband. I didn't want to end this way. I didn't want my life to end.

Tears flowed, and finally, agonizing prayer poured out from deep within me. "Lord, speak to me. I cannot do this without an awareness of Your presence. Please give me a word to sustain me."

In the quiet, Bible verses came to my mind that spoke specifically and directly to my heart. Sorrowful peace began to invade my soul. I knew I could take the next step. God was with me.

My desire is for you to experience the same quiet assurance of God's presence as you walk through your journey with cancer. Each chapter of this book is set up to be read on your own timetable. You can read a chapter a day, a chapter a week, or a chapter each month. Go at the pace of your heart and your body. My hope is that you will have space to reflect, to remember the truths of God's Word and His character, to celebrate the joys and triumphs, to grieve the sorrows, and, most of all, to remember God's faithfulness at each step.

1

HURRY UP AND SLOW DOWN

*"It's not how you die that makes the important impression, Comfort,
it's how you live. Now go live awhile."*
—*Each Little Bird That Sings,* Deborah Wiles

*H*ere you are: in a place you never thought you would be and never wanted to be, having to face the unknown one step at a time. The journey is yours, but it affects every person who knows about your battle with cancer. In this little book are some of the issues that don't usually get addressed as you walk this road. I am praying your heart will be encouraged and better prepared for the road ahead. Here's how my journey began.

Several years prior to my diagnosis with Stage II breast cancer, I picked up Rick Warren's *The Purpose Driven Life.* To be perfectly honest, I only decided to read it because my friends were reading it. My bored attitude could easily be summed up: "Ho-hum, another fix-it-in-forty-days manual, complete with simplistic answers!" However, by the time I reached day six, I was hooked.

Day six emphasizes two facts: 1) Life is brief. 2) Earth is a temporary residence. Warren ends the chapter with a question: "How should the fact that life is temporary change the way I'm living right now?"

Now I ask you, how is a person supposed to answer that in only one day? I could not stop thinking about it. So, rather than rush through it, I decided to concentrate on day six until I answered it to my own satisfaction.

My churning mind drove me to reflect on our annual trip to see my folks in Maine. Each time we go, I witness the changes in my aging parents, and I watch my nieces and nephews graduate, get married, and start their families. As I soak it all in, I feel the chilling awareness of life's brevity pierce my heart like a cold north wind on a winter's day. I turn and face my own children. As if in a time-lapsed photo, I watch in awe as they unfold like roses reaching for the sun.

Two answers for Rick Warren's question come to me. The first answer is that I must change my life by adding urgency to it.

The people I rub shoulders with every day have spiritual needs. These are the people God allows me to influence. My time with them is my opportunity to express His love through my words and my actions. The clock is ticking. I need to pray with passion and extend myself to others because my life (or theirs) may end soon.

Is my friend discouraged? Will the grocery bagger remember God's love because of me? Will I risk rejection because I love my neighbors enough to broach the topic of what will happen to them after they die? Do my children know I love them? Have I spoken encouraging words to cheer on my husband as he faces his daily routine?

People all around me are desperate for hope and desperate to know they are loved and their lives have significance. Life is temporary. That fact ought to add urgency to the way I engage with the people around me.

The second part of my answer to Warren's question is that I should change my life by savoring each day. The truth is that today is all I have on this earth. This moment with these children, friends, or strangers is given to me today. Cherishing the aroma of a baby's sweet-sour smell; internally empathizing with the pouty face of a thwarted eight-year-old; fully engaging my heart during the passionate discourse of a budding teenager—each moment is to be handled and savored as though it is eternally significant . . . because it is. These vignettes of experiences are the stuff of life for me and for those with whom I interact. The fleeting nature of life burns within me the realization that I need to hurry up and slow down.

What about you? You have been slowed down by cancer. It may seem unlikely right now, but you will have time to reflect on your life as you cope with the disease. I want to encourage you to use this time to hurry up and slow down. Go ahead and assess your spiritual health. Take an honest look inside yourself. No one lives forever. This is your opportunity to set your feet on solid ground by dealing with these ultimate issues. Capitalize on the experience so that you may reap the full benefits available to both your body and your soul.

Anticipate and set your attention on those moments that need to be savored. Linger over them. Allow the urgency of the moment to help you put away petty issues or confront broken situations so you can be free to treasure and enjoy time well spent with those closest to you. This is your invitation to hurry up and slow down!

BIBLE VERSES TO READ

- ☐ Psalm 56:3

- ☐ Jeremiah 29:11

- ☐ 1 Peter 1:7

- ☐ 1 Peter 5:7

- ☐ Psalm 139:1-18

REFLECTIONS

In the quiet of your heart, listen to God speak through these verses. Write down which verse encourages you the most and why. Which verse challenges you the most? Why?

What does Psalm 139:1-18 say about God's awareness of you?

In what ways can you discern God preparing for your needs now? List any of your needs about which you feel unsure how they will be met.

WEEK IN REVIEW

This week's high:

This week's low:

List the names of those who loved you well this week and share a brief description of what they did.

WEEK IN REVIEW

Today I feel . . .

My favorite quote this week is . . .

My favorite Bible verse this week is . . .

JOURNAL PROMPTS

How would you like to slow down and enjoy moments and people during the next few months? What moments are you hoping to enjoy? Which people?

Record your diagnosis story and your feelings surrounding it.

How are you feeling about God in this moment? How do your feelings compare to what the Scripture says is true of God? What will it look like for you to intentionally follow the Lord on this journey, no matter the outcome?

MY PRAYERS THIS WEEK

2

MIRROR-IMAGE MERCY

"I come from a family with a lot of dead people."
—Ten-year-old Comfort in Each Little Bird That Sings

S hortly before my journey with cancer began, my husband, Roger, and I were enjoying a quiet Saturday morning. Slowly rocking in mindless reverie, Roger looked over at our lone goldfish and said contentedly, with a half-smile, "The life of a goldfish . . ."

Like a shot out of nowhere, I spat back at him, "Destined to die—just like everything else is."

My heart felt restless and my stomach churned. Over several weeks, my anguish had been steadily growing. Death hung heavy around me like a dark, foreboding shadow. A childhood friend's young wife was dying from breast cancer. His sister just found out she had hepatitis C, and the impending need for a liver transplant loomed in her future. My brother's dear friend underwent surgery for a brain tumor. My cousin's husband, diagnosed with cancer, had only a year to live.

These friends had not led long and full lives. They had not yet fulfilled the hopes and dreams of their hearts. These were young people with children to nurture. Their lives were not lived. This should not be happening! My heart screamed, "Stop! Turn this horror show off. Let me walk out of this dark theater into the light once again." But the light didn't come.

My cousin's letter about her husband's cancer included two phrases that reduced me to tears. "Donne, I don't understand. I don't want him to go." In those two short sentences lay all the deepest makings of human vulnerability. The truth is that we are helpless to control the times and events of our lives. We cannot see the future or even begin to control our ultimate destiny.

I remember the first time I felt this sucking whirlpool of helplessness. I was sitting in the front row during a Bible conference holding our three-month-old baby girl. I could not keep my eyes off of her, afraid I would miss some slight pink movement. I was drinking her in—as could only a woman who married late and was told the natural course of pregnancy would not happen—and then it did! Life came forth from my body and blossomed before my very eyes into brown-haired perfection.

Through the haze of my wonder, the speaker's voice rang in my ears. "It is appointed unto man once to die . . ." A suffocating terror gripped my soul. I couldn't protect my sweet baby girl from life's ultimate end. She, too, would one day stop breathing, and her life would be over. Despite all the love and protection I could provide, I could not stop it from happening to her.

I wonder if God felt the same when His only Son entered time and history. His Son, too, would be subject to death. God the Father, all powerful and all loving, willfully did not protect Jesus from the cross. All the intensity of His thirty-three years of life did not stop the clock from ticking—nor did it stop His destiny with death. He had to face it by Himself. When Jesus asked for the circumstances of His death to be changed, the Father denied His only Son this one desperate request. The very heavens closed in a vise grip that spiraled Jesus down, down, down to face death alone. The Heir to Glory died. He left behind a grieving mother, bereft friends, and unlived years of life. He was cut down in the prime of His life. And God did not stop it.

You all know the story. Three long, sad days later, some grieving friends went to the tomb to finish the task of embalming Him. Through the mist of their tears and the morning fog, they discovered an empty tomb.

To their astounded hearts, hope burst forth as an angel declared, "He is not here. He is risen" (Matthew 28:6). Could it be? Jesus alive? Death is not the final destiny! Then, with their very eyes, they saw the risen Son of God. He spoke to them, ate with them, and reminded them of things that were once mysterious but, now, in the aura of His very presence, crystallized into stunning reality. His death assured resurrection to life. The hope of life after death resonated so deeply within Jesus's followers that many of them willingly died for Him rather than shrink back into the safety of denial. They did not cling to their physical bodies because they now knew death was not the worst thing. Death was not the end. Death was not their final destination. They saw Jesus. They knew He was Living Truth. They, too, would be resurrected into eternal life.

Like we do, the disciples initially wanted trivial rewards. In turn, Jesus gave them so much more. They wanted political peace, racial respect, and material security. They expected Jesus to give it to them in the ordinary way of human beings: war, laws, and Wall Street. At the end of their lives, they wanted to gloat, "I was right about Him." They would have had their peace, their freedom, and their daily bread in abundance. They could have sat around their living rooms with fat, round bellies and reminisced about the battles and the good old days. Then they would have died—just like everyone else. But like a secret message written in backward script, the mirror image of Jesus exploded their puny, temporary desire into deep, abundant life.

To this day, Jesus continues this pattern and handles things backwards to our natural way of doing things. Instead of war, He conquers hearts with love, one by one, day by day, change by willful change. As to racial respect, He brings dignity to all, uniting His people under their new identity as brothers and sisters in His family. As for material things, well, the Bible promises earthly images of such immense eternal wealth that even those who have everything in this life will realize they had nothing. Jesus offers what we all long for—deeper and wider and longer and higher.

Often, He does it by denying our fervent requests for lesser things. Then He gives us the very same thing in its eternal form within the scope of what He knows to be our greatest good.

Sometimes our needs, problems, or illnesses push our priorities back in our face so we can order them aright and finally figure out what we really want. When the heart is in tune to its own raw desire, unfettered by the trappings of mortality, its Creator has an incredible opportunity to fill it.

What is it that we truly want? Life? Purpose and meaning? Joy? Fullness and satisfaction? Is it true that these can be had in this life? Is it true that they can be had in the next life? We have a good Father. He will not give us sticks when we ask for bread (Matthew 7:9-11). You have safety to ask for what you want, so take a step back and remember to trust that He who made you will, out of His abundant goodness, give you what is the greatest good.

If He who sees the beginning from the end chooses to deny you, you can count on Him working to give you something far better. Like the daddy who says no to a twenty-five-cent ride outside Walmart in order to catch a plane to Disney World, our Father loves to give us the best gifts. What's more, He doesn't leave us alone to bear the pain of the journey. He promises His very self in the middle of it. He promises grace to make it through. He promises an end to the problem, to the suffering, to the sickness. In His mirror-image kingdom, His endings are really beginnings and His "no" is simply a pathway toward an even greater "yes."

As my heart brooded over these loved ones who were suffering so deeply, I audaciously asked the Lord to heal them. And I ask that for you, too—a long, healthy life. But I want to use this written space to ask questions that will help you face the most important eternal issues. Dare I intrude from my temporarily safe haven of health to hold your tear-stained face in my hands and ask . . . have you made peace with God? Have you understood in these crucial moments that this suffering may be mercy in disguise? Each of us must die. Many of us will rush headlong into eternity, leaving a trail of wistful wishes behind. Not all of us will stare death so bluntly in the face and be able to prepare ourselves for eternity: to grieve the undone things, to say the unsaid, to assure our loved ones of our approval, to make amends with our enemies.

Could cancer be used in the hands of a good God to give us the opportunity to deal with issues head on? Could this be a kind of upside-down mercy from the King of the mirror-image Kingdom? Could it be mercy to have the false veneer of health removed? Could it be mercy to reflect and muse on the ultimate truth and finally come to grips with it? Could it be mercy to trust in what you cannot see when the unknowns of cancer engulf you?

Surely it is mercy to be reminded that God's Son faced death, too. He conquered it that we might be resurrected into eternal life. Death, conquered by Christ, now offers Christians a pathway to experience the fullest riches of God's kingdom, far beyond our ability to even imagine. Is that not ultimately mercy?

Life: sexually transmitted and always fatal

Every day, someone dies. Every day, someone faces death. But it's not us. It's not me. Cancer brings us face to face with the reality of our vulnerability. To some degree, we feel in control of our destiny. Cancer wipes that out with six neon letters. In the middle of the night, when the stillness settles in, there's no hiding from the fact that we are going to die. Up until this point, death has been a vague, far-off possibility. "I'll probably die like my ninety-six-year-old grandmother, or I might die in an automobile accident, or I might die . . ." Those thoughts come randomly to the healthy person. Cancer moves that reality front and center, up close and personal.

King Solomon writes in Ecclesiastes 7:2: "It is better to spend your time at funerals than at parties. After all, everyone dies—so the living should take this to heart." I'm not sure I hold to the king's methods, but I agree with his point. Most of us will outlive cancer, but all will die sooner or later. What do you believe about death and life? This affects our daily lives. If we believe we will escape death, we ignore the voices that remind us we will all fall victim one day. If we believe we are little more than animals with no eternal soul, we follow our baser inclinations. If we believe we will be reincarnated, we live nicely so we will return in a better state of being. If we believe good deeds will earn us a spot in heaven, we do what we think God wants us to do. The question is of truth and faith. What is the basis of the belief system by which we live?

Throughout the Bible, bit by bit, God reveals His character. He is good. He is fearfully and frighteningly holy. He is all powerful. He is love. With that said, in the midst of life going full tilt, He tells us death is imminent and to expect it. If you have not studied the Bible, I suggest you take each step one at a time. Use a Bible in a modern translation (the NLT, NIV, and CSB are all great options) to keep the vocabulary as close as possible to the language you normally speak.

BIBLE VERSES TO READ

☐ Psalm 136

☐ Colossians 1:15

☐ Isaiah 55:8-9

☐ Psalm 18:30-36

REFLECTIONS

List the character qualities of God revealed in the verses on the previous page.

How might reflecting on God's character help you trust Him on your hardest days?

When you don't trust God, when you don't trust that His ways are perfect and better than your own, how can you respond in a healthy way to help lead your heart back toward Jesus?

WEEK IN REVIEW

This week's high:

This week's low:

List the names of those who loved you well this week and share a brief description of what they did.

WEEK IN REVIEW

Today I feel . . .

My favorite quote this week is . . .

My favorite Bible verse this week is . . .

JOURNAL PROMPTS

How can you see God's "mirror-image mercy" in your journey with cancer?

What is most difficult for you to trust about God today?

Describe and reflect on a time when you were keenly aware of God's presence with you. How might that experience give you courage for today?

MY PRAYERS THIS WEEK

3

REDEMPTION

*W*hen you entered the home where my five siblings and I grew up, you stepped into a long hallway that protected the kitchen from the icy blasts of Maine's cold, winter winds. On either side were two doors—one leading into the cool darkness of the attached barn and the other leading into the bright, noisy chaos of home. Beneath the coats hanging on the wall sat a beaten-up wicker laundry basket filled to varying degrees with recyclable soda cans. It was one of my mother's attempts to pinch pennies.

That wicker basket often became the center of a hilarious scene. At about nine years old, my younger brother began to tell jokes and develop muscles (sort of). One of his favorite exhibitions was going to the wicker basket to demonstrate to his captive audience of cynical sisters his amazing can-crushing abilities. He would roll up his sleeves and flex a little bubble of a muscle, and then slowly, with teeth clenching and World Wrestling Federation grunts, he would squeeze the can until it was a shapeless, unrecognizable lump of aluminum. Then, with glee, he would look up for our laughing approval, open the door, and chuck the can back into the wicker basket before swaggering off in pride.

Occasionally, it fell on me, as the newest driver in the bunch, to load up that wicker basket full of sticky, crumpled cans and take it to the recycling center. As I drove into the gravel yard, the sign in big, block, red letters seemed to yell—REDEMPTION CENTER. To paraphrase, the essence of Merriam-Webster's definition of redemption is buying back that which once belonged to the purchasers. At the recycling center, the bottlers actually bought back their own cans. I was pretty skeptical that anyone would pay me money for these useless scraps of metal, but I was sent on a mission, so I pushed open the door. I walked in timidly, expecting the gruff woman behind the counter to snarl at me as she took the cans. But, to my amazement, she whistled and chatted and puffed on her cigarette as she lined up the cans. To her eyes, these cans were worth what she was paying me. They had value. They could be remade and refilled.

To one degree or another, every person in the world is a crumpled lump of aluminum in God's eyes. Each one of us is crushed and victimized by the sin of others and the brokenness of the world. We have made our own sinful choices, too. For most of us, life has moments of terrifying confusion and chaos. Some of us are very much aware of our brokenness. Others more easily conceal their dents and bumps.

But each one of us needs the same redemption. Christ's redemption not only buys us back from a ruined life but liberates us from the baggage of brokenness. And that incredibly good news is just one part of the package! We can have the very source of renewed life within us! The death of Jesus Christ bought us back by paying the penalty God demanded for our sins. By His death, the lives of those who placed themselves in His care have His redemption stamped all over them—valuable, remade, filled with the Living Water. His resurrection is proof He has the power required to fulfill what may seem to us a hopeless and endless task.

In a simultaneous process of healing, molding, and filling, Christ's redemption transforms broken lives into overflowing springs, offering hope to others along the way. Just as those badly damaged cans were ultimately melted down and completely changed, we, too, are in the process of growing more and more into the image of the Great Redeemer.

Sometimes the process is heated and sometimes it is cooled, but always it is overseen by the One who never overlooks a detail or misses an opportunity to love us.

Where are you? Do you need redemption? Are you discouraged and overwhelmed by the daunting assignment facing you? The next time you are tempted to discouragement, remember that chatting, whistling recycling lady who saw value in crumpled aluminum. You are more than a body ill with cancer. God can take whatever you give Him and remake you, filling you with Living Water. Redemption includes deliverance. You are valuable. You can be remade. Living Water is waiting for you.

BIBLE VERSES TO READ

☐   Hebrews 9:15

☐   John 10:10

☐   Psalm 130:7

☐   Romans 5:10

☐   1 Corinthians 1:30

☐   1 Peter 1:18-19

REFLECTIONS

List the character qualities of God revealed in the verses on the previous page.

Romans 5:10 tells us that we are saved through the life of Jesus. How does Jesus's life save you—beyond eternal salvation? How does His life impact your daily life?

How does the truth of redemption impact the way you think about your cancer journey?

WEEK IN REVIEW

This week's high:

This week's low:

List the names of those who loved you well this week and share a brief description of what they did.

WEEK IN REVIEW

Today I feel . . .

My favorite quote this week is . . .

My favorite Bible verse this week is . . .

JOURNAL PROMPTS

In what ways does redemption give you hope?

How are you struggling to trust God today?

How can you be intentional as you take your struggles to God today, to be honest with Him about all you feel and areas in which you do not trust Him?

MY PRAYERS THIS WEEK

4

TRUST GOD FOR WHAT?

*"Jesus's death wasn't to free us from dying but to free us from the fear of death.
Jesus came to liberate us so that we could die up front and then live."*
—The Barbarian Way, Erwin McManus

*H*ave you ever heard the old proverb, "Don't be so heavenly minded that you are no earthly good"? The saying conjures up images of shallow people dreaming futile dreams and pursuing unreal visions. In contrast, real hope helps you focus on heaven and funnel your energy so your days on earth really matter.

Cancer forced me to think about heaven. My rose-colored glasses took on a gloomy, bluish tint as I sadly watched all the suffering around me. Because of my own suffering, I felt more acutely the sufferings of those around me. Elderly people whom I dearly loved seemed trapped in their aging bodies, unable to enjoy the things they loved. I saw children walking around with turbans on their bald heads and IV lines attached to rolling infusion machines. I listened to tragedy after tragedy. My heart waited in dreaded anticipation to hear about the next accident, the next illness, and the next death.

Life no longer felt full of promise. It felt full of pain and death and hurt. All my goals seemed senseless in the light of impending death. Somewhere, in the midst of my bleak fog, my perspective began to shift from wishing I could escape the suffering to wondering if my life would really matter in eternity. That question pushed me to come to grips with what I really believe about heaven. I began to picture with increasing clarity what it would be like to grasp the biblical promise of heaven while living fully in the present moment.

The guiding hope of the believer is the assurance of an eternal place in the very Presence of the Creator. This hope gives purpose for the days of our lives on earth. Every answered prayer, every met need, and every crisis weathered adds to the assurance of God's loving and intimate involvement in our lives. Hope becomes a strong network of events pointing to heaven. Where God is, hope lives.

I imagine hope to be a lot like surfboarding—the exhilarating triumph of gliding across that slippery surface of water grows into practiced confidence with each successful attempt. There are a few basic surfboarding lessons and techniques, but each wave is a new experience. Just as each new wave brings specific challenges and nuances, each situation in your life can challenge hope with a new set of problems and doubts. Every circumstance shares similar elements, but each one has unique challenges we must face as we trust God. Cancer brings a whole set of new and frightening challenges that seem as overwhelming as a tsunami. Hope may flounder in a sea of despair. Standing up and staying on the "surfboard of hope" becomes the difficult and seemingly impossible priority to stay afloat.

What exactly are we hoping for? Biblical hope is defined as confident expectancy (Hebrews 11:1). Expectancy for what? Expectancy for the Living God to enter into our circumstances and breathe His very life into them, giving us Himself and, therefore, life. I submit that the very basis of hope is life. Being faced with a negative diagnosis shakes the foundation of hope. It showed me that despite all my training in Bible college, I had only been hoping in this life. Now was the time to look beyond the temporal situations and into eternity.

Facing my own mortality helped me see that the end of this life is only a breath away for every human being. We are all subject to illnesses. No one escapes everything. No one gets out of this alive! We will not live on this earth forever. Nor would we want to. Who would want to live forever in a body subject to illness and decay? I long to encourage you to walk with Him, to get your feet firmly planted in the hope of the gospel and take each step through your whole life journey, from this day forward, experiencing Him in each situation until you are swept into His arms for eternity.

Hope is taking on a different definition for me. I no longer limit hope to getting a good parking space or winning my daily war with clutter. Hope is becoming an overarching, guiding light as I learn to carefully choose the things I am involved in and the way I live my life. If heaven is real, the choices I make can impact eternity for the better. This suffering is temporary. It will not last forever or be the end of me. My life, with cancer or without, is eternally significant and meaningful even if today is my last day on earth.

As you face your own battle with cancer, I cannot tell you why you have this disease. Our bodies are subject to death. We live in a broken world. Those realities cause immense suffering and unanswerable questions. I can, however, offer you hope that God is in control. He looks over your life with love and tenderness. He longs to respond to your need and to reveal His glory in your circumstances. I want to tenderly remind you that no one has total control of their life. This uncontrollable thing that has happened to you did not catch God by surprise. Somehow, someway, He is involved in this. And where God is, hope lives.

BIBLE VERSES TO READ

- ☐ 1 Peter 5:10

- ☐ Isaiah 40:31

- ☐ Hebrews 11:1

- ☐ Philippians 1:6

- ☐ Romans 5:5

- ☐ Romans 15:13

REFLECTIONS

List the character qualities of God revealed in the verses on the previous page.

How do these verses describe the connection between hope and the Holy Spirit?

How can the Holy Spirit help you when you lose sight of hope?

WEEK IN REVIEW

This week's high:

This week's low:

List the names of those who loved you well this week and share a brief description of what they did.

WEEK IN REVIEW

Today I feel . . .

My favorite quote this week is . . .

My favorite Bible verse this week is . . .

JOURNAL PROMPTS

Worldly hope is fleeting and without substance. Biblical hope is rooted in the faithfulness of God. What kind of hope do you think you have today?

What aspects of biblical hope are hard for you to connect to real-life circumstances?

How can you take a step toward placing your hope in God?

MY PRAYERS THIS WEEK

5

HOPE FOR HEALING

God heals. He did it in the Old Testament. He did it in the New Testament. He does it every day. He made our bodies with healing mechanisms that are astoundingly complex and wonderful. He heals instantaneously, He heals through processes, and He heals through medicine. He gave us minds to figure out how things work and allows us to be in on the healing process through science and medicine. He gives gifts of healing to the church to bring healing into our lives supernaturally. He gives Himself to us for miraculous healing.

We can legitimately look to Him with hope for healing. Ask. Listen for His leading and follow Him in openness and submission in every aspect of your life. I believe true healing encompasses our whole being—not just our bodies. Heaven is a place of complete and full healing in every area of our beings.

We are body, spirit, and soul. Are there emotional or soul wounds in your life that need to be healed? Are there relationships that need mending? Are there sin issues you need to address? In your desperation for physical healing, do not overlook these areas. They could be even more important than your physical well-being.

God heals in different ways. He promises in James 1:5 that He will give us wisdom and guidance if we ask for it. Ask Him about your treatment plan. Be careful to listen for Him to give you peace and assurance as you follow in obedience. As that process is at work, He promises grace to face the next step. But do not hesitate to ask God for physical healing. You have a good Father who loves to give you good gifts.

Your health is intimately tied up with God's purpose for your life and for the lives of those with whom you interact. God heals to validate His supremacy. He heals to encourage our faith and the faith of those who need to believe. He heals because there is great need. He heals because He is moved by compassion. He heals because He sovereignly appoints it. He heals because He is the Healer. He heals because He loves us. He heals so that more people may know, love, and honor Him. He heals for reasons we cannot comprehend.

You may be rolling your eyes, nodding toward gravestones of loved ones who were not healed. God, in His infinite wisdom and goodness, does not heal all physical illness. God uses every circumstance. He lovingly matures our character and faith through the difficulties and blessings of our lives. He uses suffering as part of that maturing process.

Every human being suffers to some degree. The difference is that the suffering of believers need never be in vain. In the study *Believing God*, Beth Moore writes, "As we allow God to minister to us in our fiery trials, He is glorified, the church is edified, and we are qualified for greater reward."

James 4:2 says, "You have not because you ask not." My job is to encourage you to ask. You have no guarantees in this life without Jesus. In His wisdom, for our good, He very seldom tells us the future. He wants us to trust Him with the unknown. He wants us to exercise faith that He might prove Himself faithful and be experientially known by you.

Moore's study, *Believing God*, has been a tremendous comfort and help in my life. Through that video series, she helped me understand how God's love can be expressed in the way he chooses to heal.

She writes: "I wonder whether the way He heals may vary according to His objective.

If the primary objective is to show His supremacy, (for instance, accreditation), perhaps He might choose to heal instantaneously. If His primary objective is to teach sufficiency in Him or to mature and build faith, I would wonder whether He heals through a stitch-by-stitch method. Remember God is far more interested in our knowing the Healer than He is in the healing. God can be vastly glorified through either objective; showing His supremacy or His sufficiency."

We experience God's sufficiency through grace. As my treatment began to wind down, the effects were more severe. Two of my sisters told me they could come from Maine for a week to help out. Somehow, I knew that the next-to-the-last treatment would be a doozy. I asked them to come at that time. To this day, I know that they were the physical embodiment of God's enabling power and His sufficiency for me for that treatment. I was so dreading the chemo that I know I would have hidden under the bed rather than drive to the clinic.

My sisters arrived at my house late in the afternoon the day before that treatment. We laughed and visited, and then they went to bed. The next day, they took over the morning routine and whisked the kids out the door. Before I had time to realize what was happening, they nudged and prodded me into my clothes and out the door. We were at the clinic and I was hooked up before I could even protest. Patti kept me laughing while Sis instinctively fixed the bed and covered me up. The next thing I knew, I was drugged and at home lying in bed. They were the enabling power of God when I lacked the courage and will to do the next thing.

I know there is available grace for each treatment, each decision, each encounter, and each step of the way you must take. As in anything that is offered, you must reach out for it to grab hold of it. Pour out your heart, listen to God, and allow Him to answer and fill you with His grace. This moment-by-moment awareness and openness of your spirit to the movement of the Holy Spirit is a level of commitment beyond mental assent of biblical truths. It requires a commitment to put God first in your life no matter the cost. It involves opening yourself up to Him in total vulnerability.

How will God work? That's like the joke about the elephant. "When an elephant goes out to the movies, where does he sit?" The answer: "Anywhere he likes!" How will God work? Anyway He chooses.

The Scriptures do not give us a prescription for God's healing decisions, but they do make His character known. No matter His choice, you can rest assured it will be done for your good out of the utmost love of His heart. God is the Creator of the Universe. He speaks and worlds are formed. He is the God of Abraham, Isaac, and Jacob. He is intimately interested in each individual life He creates. He is the One who takes shepherd boys and makes them kings! He is the God of love and justice all rolled into One and nailed on a cross. He is the God who raises the dead to life! He is also the God who chastises when His children sin, who throws parties for prodigals, and who uses the empires of the world for His sovereign plans.

How will He work in your life? That's part of the adventure you are called to witness as you walk with Him through this journey. Open your heart, open your hands, and rest in His love.

BIBLE VERSES TO READ

☐ Mark 4:35-41; the power of Jesus over _____

☐ Mark 5:1-20; the power of Jesus over _____

☐ Mark 5:21-34; the power of Jesus to _____

☐ Mark 5:35-43; the power of Jesus over _____

☐ James 4:2; 5:14-16

☐ John 9:1-33

REFLECTIONS

What does Jesus have power over? Does that include your illness?

Have you specifically asked Him to heal you? Have you asked the elders to anoint you with oil and pray over you? Will you? If you have, record the date, the names, and all you can remember.

How could your situation bring glory to the name of Jesus? Are you expecting Him to be honored through this life experience ?

WEEK IN REVIEW

This week's high:

This week's low:

List the names of those who loved you well this week and share a brief description of what they did.

WEEK IN REVIEW

Today I feel . . .

My favorite quote this week is . . .

My favorite Bible verse this week is . . .

JOURNAL PROMPTS

Do you have trouble trusting the Lord for healing in this life? In this situation?

Do you have a sense of how He might heal your body from cancer? Describe it.

If you could tell others a story of how Jesus has sustained you in this trial, what would you say to them? Can you list ways that He has met your needs?

MY PRAYERS THIS WEEK

6

RISING TO THE OCCASION

"Mama dabbed at my face with a Snowberger's handkerchief. 'Uncle Edisto always said, "It takes courage to look life in the eye and say yes to"—what did he call it?' 'The messy glory,' I said."
—Each Little Bird That Sings

*a*bout a week before Christmas, I went on a field trip with Michael's second-grade class to the movies. We saw *Mr. Magorium's Wonder Emporium.* It is the story of a young and beautiful composer, Molly Mahoney, who works in a toy store. Her boss, Mr. Magorium, who is played by Dustin Hoffman, tells her he is leaving. When it dawns on her that he means he is going to die, she refuses to accept it. He explains that he has done what he could and what he was supposed to do. Now it is her turn to run the store. She protests. Holding her face tenderly in his hands, he looks into her eyes and says, "Your life is an occasion. Rise to it."

When the doctor told me that I had cancer, it felt more like a death sentence than an occasion. Was God really allowing me to go through this? My life verse is Philippians 3:10: "I want to know Christ and the power of His resurrection and the fellowship of sharing in His sufferings, becoming like Him in His death . . ."

Could God use cancer to further my experience of Him and give me a deeper understanding and connection to His sufferings? Well, here I was. The diagnosis was clear and undeniable. There was no way out of it. No reverse. No rewind. The question hanging before my heart in brilliant flashing neon was: would I walk with Him through this?

The Bible tells us in Psalm 34:17, "The righteous face many troubles, but the Lord rescues them from each and every one." Troubles are the very stage God uses to display His goodness to a world full of people walking on a journey toward death. Even cancer is a stage God uses for His good purposes.

When I picked up my head and looked at my children watching me, I wanted them to know that, even in cancer, God is faithful. They needed to experience His goodness in this trial, too. Who knows what lies ahead for each of them? This was one more occasion for the Lord to strengthen their trust. It was also one more occasion for me to experience the reality of the Living God in my life. Like a four-year-old child, I mentally put my hand in His and took the next step. Enabled by God, the human soul is created to rise up and tackle the challenges life brings us, even cancer. I didn't feel electrical impulses charging through my body, but I did feel peace, and I was able to rise and do the next thing.

Despite all the variations of personality, environment, temperament, and taste in each individual soul, no person is outside the scope and sweep of God's plan and ability to enable and rescue. There is never a circumstance beyond His power to change. I believe that includes cancer. I believe that includes you. But we cannot responsibly bask in the comfort of that truth without stepping out in faith to grapple with the realities that cancer raises in our lives. Those realities—needs, fears, and unknowns—make up the nitty-gritty situation that is our occasion. We do not know what effect our lives will have on those watching. This is one more opportunity to allow the Lord to use your life. Steward the days and opportunities. Rise.

In the Bible, there is a book about an orphaned girl, Esther, who saves the day for the Jewish people. Esther faced the ultimate call of stewardship. Her uncle, Mordecai, pointed out to her that the very reason for her existence might culminate in this one historic moment. With a trembling heart and empty stomach, she laid herself open to God in a three-day fast. Then she rose to the occasion and history was changed. Lives were saved. God moved. Jesus was born through the line of Judah. Eternity was effected.

We don't know what our ultimate call of stewardship will be, but we do know that each day, there are opportunities before us to follow Esther's example, believe God is with us, and expect Him to act. Don't you long for that soul-satisfying knowledge that your life really matters? I know I do. God is asking you to trust Him in this time of your life. Rise to the occasions God brings to you, steward well the events and blessings of your life, and taste the goodness of a God who rescues the righteous from their many troubles.

BIBLE VERSES TO READ

- ☐ Philippians 3:10

- ☐ Psalm 34:17

- ☐ Esther 4:14b

- ☐ Psalm 23

- ☐ Psalm 27:1, 13-14

- ☐ Book of Esther

REFLECTIONS

Philippians 3:10 is a commitment that in every circumstance, knowing Jesus through experiencing Him is the goal of life. What ways can you know Him in your suffering with cancer? How can you draw near to Him?

(Psalm 34:17) Make a list of possible ways God can deliver you from your situation.

Esther's occasion that she chose to rise for concluded in the salvation of God's plan of redemption for the world. Imagine all the good your rising in trust and obedience to God in this situation could bring to the world around you.

WEEK IN REVIEW

This week's high:

This week's low:

List the names of those who loved you well this week and share a brief description of what they did.

WEEK IN REVIEW

Today I feel . . .

My favorite quote this week is . . .

My favorite Bible verse this week is . . .

JOURNAL PROMPTS

What is the most difficult thing your treatment has required of you?

What is the most difficult thing God has asked you to do as you receive treatment? What makes it hard to rise to this challenge?

(Psalm 27:1, 13-14) Take a few minutes and write out these verses in your own words. Shout them out loud and affirm that you are certain to see the Lord's goodness in the land of the living. Then write down three ways God has revealed His goodness to you this week.

MY PRAYERS THIS WEEK

7

PICKING UP THE PIECES

"Sometimes I ask him (my daddy) how somebody died. He tells me; then he says,
'It's not how you die that makes the important impression, Comfort; it's how you live.
Now go live awhile, honey, and let me get back to work.' "
—*Each Little Bird That Sings*

I have long been plagued with a Cinderella-type illusion. It goes like this: all the mean-spirited people in my life will get their just due, and I, in my own little corner, will be cherished and reign in the end. It plays out to mean nothing more than that I will have a smoothly running household with children who agree with me without terrible conflict. My husband will dote on me. I will be a svelte size eight with abs and biceps. I will be able to accomplish every responsibility on time and with top-notch quality. I will glide from one PTA meeting to another while attending soccer games in between.

All the while, I will nurture my friends and family as only I know how. The house will run like clockwork, with everyone doing their chores without being reminded because they want to do them! The dog's hair will fall out outside instead of on the rug in the living room. We will have enough money to say no to the children because it's not good for them to have too much instead of saying no because we don't have money for the brands they like. Life will be smooth and even-keeled. God will bless our family and keep us from pain and hurt.

Your response is likely similar to the common response of my sixteen-year-old: "Good luck with that!"

As I gradually settled back into a chaotic routine, I began to see that life would never be the same again. I was physically unable to keep up with my responsibilities. Cancer treatment took a toll on my body. I could no longer mask my procrastination with frenzied activity. The way I used to live no longer worked. This realization was not a pretty experience. It became clearer than ever that my illusion was an unattainable, unrealistic, nebulous fantasy. Reality tells me that life is not ever going to be like that for anyone for very long. Life is tough and has its challenges. I couldn't make my dream come true.

I soon felt like I was drowning in the chaos of increasing responsibilities and decreasing resources. For weeks, I muddled through, trying to keep up with my routine. Despair often overtook me as my failure to keep up became blatantly obvious. I hurt the children with my uncontrolled tongue and overindulgence. I blamed my husband for minor infractions to shift the blame and prove the difficulties in my life were his fault. If he would just change and do things my way for once, my life would make sense.

Shame and accusation surrounded my every thought. I could not escape. No one called me. I felt like my dearest cousin grew tired of hearing me whine and blame. All my friends seemed to sense my overflowing cesspool of need and were too busy to help. My husband no longer wanted to enter the whirlwind with me. I couldn't blame any of them. I was tired of me, too.

Finally, in desperation, I laid my soul bare before God. I felt adrift and abandoned as I kept the schedule rolling with meals, laundry, bake sales, carpooling, piano lessons, soccer practice, house cleaning, checking on aging parents, dog shots, fighting the insurance company, and getting the trees that border our property cut down. I wept at the pain I inflicted on my daughter. I saw with clarity how my grace giving had contributed to sin on the part of another child. I failed to come through on several things for a third child. I missed important moments and exciting discoveries because I overscheduled. I could no longer satiate my thirsty soul using someone else's resources or deny the truth that I had been trying to use someone else's answers to meet the crying need of my heart. I couldn't hide it from myself any longer. The truth was that my fairytale illusion did not serve me well and did not hold up under the stresses I faced. My life was in pieces and I couldn't make it fit anymore.

My heart broke. I found myself truly apologizing for hurting my husband. I gave him fewer reasons for my actions and felt more concern for his life. I began to put myself in the shoes of my children. I could feel my verbal assault as I tried to get them to conform to what I desired. The pain of the truth helped me change my tactics. I tried standing firm when I said no. I began trying to reach their hearts instead of controlling their schedules and lives. I saw the need to require responsibility rather than demand perfection. Gradually, other areas and relationships in my life started taking on a new shape. I am not the same person anymore.

This is really different and it is coming from a place deep within me that has never before been allowed to surface. When did this begin? The trauma of cancer and the grace of God intermingled to offer me the pathway to freedom from self. Like someone waking up from a long sleep, I shook off the dream. This is my reality. This is where God wants me—in this moment, for these children, with this man, living out the truth of God's Word in the midst of the struggles that life brings and the residue of cancer and its treatment. God wants to be real to me in this moment. Today. Right now. That is what picking up the pieces has been all about for me. What will it be for you?

BIBLE VERSES TO READ

☐ Ephesians 1:18-19

☐ Romans 8:31-36

☐ Romans 12:1-2

☐ Romans 8:28-30

REFLECTIONS

(Ephesians 1:17-19) What circumstances do you foresee needing wisdom for as you progress into the next stage of healing? Whom can you depend upon to guide you and help you?

(Romans 8:31-36) According to this passage, what is able to stand against God's children?

(Romans 12:1-2) What do you need to transform in your way of thinking about your current circumstances to put them into the proper perspective according to these verses?

WEEK IN REVIEW

This week's high:

This week's low:

List the names of those who loved you well this week and share a brief description of what they did.

WEEK IN REVIEW

Today I feel . . .

My favorite quote this week is . . .

My favorite Bible verse this week is . . .

JOURNAL PROMPTS

Take a few minutes and talk to the Lord about this aspect of your life that He has allowed.

List the things that seem to be against you at the moment and let the Scripture wash over them. Bring your thoughts about those things to be put into order according to Scripture.

What are you tempted to tell yourself about this situation? Practice doing as Romans 12:1-2 says by imagining yourself in front of the throne, offering your life to Him to use as He sees fit. Remind yourself in writing to Whom you are giving yourself.

MY PRAYERS THIS WEEK

8

WHAT IF?

*O*ne of the more difficult realities that people with cancer have to deal with is the ever-present unknown. The unknown is no longer a fuzzy, rose-colored shade. It is a dark, even sinister, shadow that hovers over the future. Even after treatment and surgery, the what-ifs linger. After all, you did not receive a grand announcement the first time cancer came around. It showed up in a sneaky, insidious invasion. What's to say it won't happen twice? Who am I to escape cancer again? Planning for the future is clouded with the possibility of another battle with this disease. Long-term goals and desires seem futile in the face of cancer's havoc. Sometimes I feel like a gerbil spinning on a wheel with the hot breath of an evil monster breathing down my neck. No matter how fast I run, it's still right there, breathing hot, stinking clouds of doom over my life.

I was blessed with a very good prognosis from the doctors' statistical standpoint. Some of you reading this might be in an altogether different situation with more serious challenges to face. Regardless of your prognosis, God's character remains unchanged.

He loves you. He sees you. And He is pursuing your heart. Your heart is God's primary concern. Sometimes, in His loving kindness, He uses your health to access the deepest places of your heart.

I wish I could offer you an easy answer on this road, but each one of us has to kneel in submission before a loving and sovereign Lord and surrender the control of our future to Him. We cannot surrender by reading a book or listening to someone else's story. While those things encourage us to believe God can heal us, they are not a substitute for our own personal engagement with God about this issue. I have found that I must repeatedly surrender control of my health until I feel peace deep within my soul.

Trusting the Lord and surrendering my health to Him is an ongoing battle. Every time the fear surfaces, I grab it by the ear and go to a quiet place to lay it out again before the Lord. My life is not my own. I am not my own. I have been bought with a price. Is this my destiny? I think not. I want to live. I ask for life. I ask if there are areas that need to be changed to conform to what God wants. I determine to obey. I place my life, my days, my health, my concerns, my loved ones, and whatever surfaces in His hands, and I listen. When my heart is satisfied that He spoke into my life again, I move on in obedience to whatever He told me to do. I write it down. I am living this day for Him. I have no more assurance of tomorrow than another person, but I do have this day, this word, this step, and I refuse to allow fear to rob me of the opportunity to experience God today.

In any circumstance in our lives, a certain amount of grieving for what used to be must take place before we can move ahead. This is particularly true with cancer. Your life will be forever different. Your body, changed by the cancer and by the treatment, will require different care. Facing such a daunting trial changes your soul, softening it to the sufferings of others and hardening it to your own sufferings, or you may wallow in the muck of self-pity and self-preservation.

I want to challenge you to surrender each day to the Lord, to give Him your very minutes and trust Him to lead you through this situation. Do not be waylaid by the muck. Take care of the issues at hand. Fear is the first one. Paint a picture of stretching out prostrate before the Lord and giving Him the rights to your life. Allow Him to have access to your heart. Ask Him to remove the fear and replace it with discernment about your body's needs. Ask Him to remind you of reality. Pray that fear will be removed from your heart, that you will face the next treatment with courage and grace with your hand in His.

If you fail and get stuck in the muck, take a nap. Try again until His hand holding yours becomes a permanent image in your mind. You are deeply loved, and God has not left you alone in this suffering. He has promised to be with us to the end. Hold Him to it.

Once fear is handled, life begins anew. There is possibility ahead at every turn instead of doom.

"Nothing can separate us from the love of God in Christ Jesus . . ." Nothing. The same God who used ten awful plagues to free the Israelites from hundreds of years of slavery can take your cancer journey and turn it into a meaningful platform for the grace of God to be revealed to you in a myriad of ways. I long for you to be free of fear and full of expectation for the revelation of God to you.

What about you? Where are you with the issue of ongoing fear?

BIBLE VERSES TO READ

- ☐ John 14:27

- ☐ Matthew 6:34

- ☐ Isaiah 43:1

- ☐ Psalm 23:4

- ☐ Romans 8:38-39

- ☐ 1 Peter 5:6-7

- ☐ Isaiah 41:10

- ☐ Isaiah 41:3

REFLECTIONS

Write your fears below. Look at them in black and white. Read all the verses on the previous page aloud and choose the ones that speak to your fear. Write them down. Memorize one verse.

What has the Lord promised you in each of these verses?

Will you let the Lord help you through fear into freedom? Write out your prayer to Him, even if you are having a hard time believing.

WEEK IN REVIEW

This week's high:

This week's low:

List the names of those who loved you well this week and share a brief description of what they did.

WEEK IN REVIEW

Today I feel . . .

My favorite quote this week is . . .

My favorite Bible verse this week is . . .

JOURNAL PROMPTS

Describe your largest battle with fear. Answer the when, where, and what questions.

Who have you told about your fear? What steps are you taking to stand against it?

What changes in your life due to cancer do you dread most?

MY PRAYERS THIS WEEK

9

SHATTERED PATHWAYS

"Uncle Edisto always said, 'Every ending is a new beginning.'"
—Each Little Bird That Sings

*H*onestly, I was trying to be understanding. I had just read a celebrity's story of struggle over leaving one high-paying job for another. On the surface, her boyfriend's perspective seemed deep and helpful. "A bend in the road is not the end of the road—if you remember to take the turn." In other words, he was saying, "Be flexible; enjoy the unexpected scenery. Even the negatives can eventually be positive." Later on, when I read the hidden anguish in an email from a dear friend, the celebrity's article turned to meaningless fluff.

Denise and I met in Italy as young missionary wives and mothers struggling through language school. Together, as only women do, we faced daily unexpected turns as we wrestled with adjusting to a new culture. Then both of our families, through a series of puzzling events, landed back in North America, stunned, confused, and wondering what to do next. As I reflected on the bend in the road our somewhat parallel lives had taken, faces of a group of women appeared in my mind. Their lives, too, took unexpected and sometimes tragic bends that left them breathless and dependent. In fact, in contrast to a meandering, winding road with pleasant, albeit unexpected, heights and depths, I would say their lives had been bombed.

Juanita faced with humor and courage the challenges of caring for her precious Elizabeth, who has brittle bone disease. Susan's mother-heart has been anguished and fought for Gordon, her son who contracted polio from a vaccine when he was a baby. Teresa lovingly shouldered the chaos and demands of her sweet husband's quadriplegia. Emily gracefully managed the ups and downs of autism with Chase. Courageously staring her own mortality in the face, Mary Jane passed the five-year marker from breast cancer. Eva, a paraplegic since age seventeen, faces her suffering honestly and is used by God in the lives of all within her reach. These situations will not change from one high road to another. The daily realities of pain and the ravages of disease face them in a grueling daily marathon. Yes, they would say that God, in His supreme goodness, has unexpected turns for each of us. But sometimes, God, in His inexplicable goodness, allows the whole road to be blown up. Smack dab ahead is a grand detour that leads into a field of land mines surrounded by snipers named doubt and insecurity.

Questions that lie dormant as we travel down normal bends in the road of life come unbidden to the surface. "Why me? Where is God in all this? Is God here? It's my fault. If only . . ." The road map of hopes and expectations has been blown up with the road. How do we cope with this? There are no signs to indicate what's up ahead, only a gut feeling that it will be hard and may never get easier. A cold, clammy death settles over the soul as the old, familiar road slips away. Images of happy homes and tranquil situations pop up in stark contrast to the messy debris of our illness. Intense longing and hopelessness come right behind those images.

In our technological age, where asking is receiving, we are programmed to want what we want when we want it. Accepting what is less than ideal is not mildly irritating or disappointing. It is enough to send us into a rage. We do not want to bend with this turn in the road. We want *our* road, and, within our souls, we raise an angry fist at a silent, unmoving ceiling.

Susan said it well one day. In her quiet, steady voice, she said, "Some of us have to learn to live with a broken heart." It is not enough to bend with the turns in our lives. We must bow because the real question is one of control. We must ultimately answer this question: who really has control of the unexpected, unplanned, unwanted tragedies in our life?

Is there really an unseen hand guiding our steps? Does our suffering have purpose and meaning? Is God in the midst of this mess, this disappointment, this paralysis, this cancer, this thing that we did not want? How can we face one more day, one more hour, and one more minute?

Those bombs that blow up our roads and send us slogging through an uncharted detour also clear the way of a lot of unnecessary debris. The illusion of self-sufficiency is usually the first to go. That "pick yourself up by your own bootstraps" mentality is replaced by a terrifying awareness of your own need. Untested theology and spiritual cockiness that lead to thoughts such as "God doesn't work that way" are wiped out and replaced, at first, by a flood of doubt and fear. Those ritualistic spiritual disciplines take on a different outlook altogether. As we teeter between anger and helplessness, those occasional spurts of prayer become a life-altering experience. Eventually, when all the shallow trappings of life are wiped away, our undefined desires for tasting great goodness are crystallized by the very thing that threatens our happiness. In the suffering, the self-denial, and the daily grind, we will finally find rest in the greatest goodness of all. Without the bomb, we would not know God as we know Him now. This is the stuff real life is made of—not some shady country lane that meanders from one pleasant scene to another. This is the stuff that calls from us character, self-discipline, and faith.

While waiting in the X-ray department to confirm yet another broken bone, Juanita's eleven-year-old, Elizabeth Shaw, recited this psalm, produced from a heart that is wise beyond her years because she daily endures suffering:

When the times are tough
I will trust in thee
Even tho' it's hard

There's nothing that can turn me
Away.
Even tho' I am feeling pain
Even tho' I cannot feel you
You are with me
Trying to comfort me
Things are hard for me
But you always stand by
Through the good and the bad
Through the worst and the best
You help me get back on my feet
In danger you keep me safe
And until it is time for me to go
Home
I will never let go.

Elizabeth caught it. Jesus alone knows how to enable us to go on until we can go Home. This journey does not come with formulas, ten-step programs, or little to-do lists. Only the very face of Jesus in the fog of pain enables us to endure. The heart of Jesus, through shared tears, gives us courage. The hands of Jesus, through an unexpected stranger, encourage our hearts. The presence of the One who intercedes for us is our provision for the road ahead. God gives us enabling grace for this minute and the next. Jesus bears our burdens and gives us strength when we are helpless. When our roads are bombed, all that remains is Jesus Himself. And He, my friends, is all that is necessary to face that next bend in the road. Through Jesus, God provides us with all we need to face the new road ahead of us.

BIBLE VERSES TO READ

☐ Mark 5:25-34

☐ Matthew 9:18-26

☐ John 6:66-69

☐ 1 Samuel 1:1-18

☐ Esther 4

REFLECTIONS

Describe how cancer has bombed your life, your plans, and your dreams.

As you are picking up the pieces of your life, what is one relationship, one issue, or one reality that you need to approach differently because of cancer?

How can pouring out your heart to God help?

WEEK IN REVIEW

This week's high:

This week's low:

List the names of those who loved you well this week and share a brief description of what they did.

WEEK IN REVIEW

Today I feel . . .

My favorite quote this week is . . .

My favorite Bible verse this week is . . .

JOURNAL PROMPTS

What has the bomb of cancer in your life blown up?

As the dust settles around you, what changes do you see ahead?

What possibilities do you see in the ashes of the losses you have suffered? Pray over this and take time to really ponder.

MY PRAYERS THIS WEEK

10

WHEN THEY DON'T COME

"He that cannot forgive others breaks the bridge over which he must pass
himself, for every man has need to be forgiven."
—*Thomas Fuller*

The responsibility for the well-being of my grandparents fell squarely on my dad's shoulders. He was the youngest of eight children and brought his bride home to his parents. We lived on the second floor of their old, Victorian-style house. When Grandmother Grant had a stroke that left her bedridden, my mother added her care to the daily routine of mothering four small children. When the time became necessary, my dad made arrangements for my grandmother to be put in a nursing home on his mail route. He made daily stops at lunchtime to visit and comfort her. His love for his mother was genuine and self-sacrificing. And in light of his deep love, he never understood the way one of his brothers reacted to their mother's illness. This brother lived out of state and would come to visit but was perpetually unable to make the detour to the nursing home to visit his mother. Years later, when Grandfather Grant had to recuperate in a nursing home for a short time, this same brother drove by the home without stopping. My dad could not fathom how anyone could be so callous and thoughtless toward their own parent.

As time passed on my journey with cancer, I grew in awareness of several people whose absence from my side screamed to me. I felt tempted to think that our friendship must not have held as much meaning as I thought. Maybe I did something to offend them. Maybe they thought I deserved this and left me to struggle alone. Perhaps they were selfish and thoughtless. Or maybe they were weak and frightened, not knowing what to say, not willing to admit their fear of loss, fear of life without me, or fear of their own vulnerability.

I feel confident that you also may experience some conspicuous absences during your illness. Even though I was overwhelmed with loving and caring help, some people just didn't come. Thankfully, early in my diagnosis, I became aware that this was not only about me, but cancer would also have effects on my family and friends. The question before me remained: would I allow God to use my suffering to do a work in the lives of my friends and family without bitterness?

I was able to let go of the pain of those absences partly because my needs were graciously cared for by loved ones but mostly because the Spirit gave me grace not to grow bitter from their absence and instead to be curious about what was going on in their hearts.

I began to look and listen more carefully to all of my friends and family members' lives. Jodi, my phone friend and confidante through many difficult times, had recently nursed and nurtured another dear friend through breast cancer—and the friend died. I didn't realize how closely involved she had been with this friend. She could not bear to see me go through it, too. She continued to call me regularly, but I didn't lay eyes on her almost the entire time I was sick. Not until my treatment ended did Jodi tell me that she wept after every phone call. At separate times, three women each confessed that their own mother died of breast cancer and the memories were so painful when they saw me that they were unable to visit again. Another acquaintance brought me a cheery fall sign that she made and shared the same story while standing on the front porch with her car running.

I suspect the issues of facing personal mortality and the vulnerability of life itself keep many from coming. Some aren't able to face their own fear. They stay away because they don't want to add another burden of fear to the cancer patient. Others are a little superstitious, and they think, "If I don't get near them, I won't get cancer."

Cancer is not a disease that affects only the patient. Every person who comes into contact with you must filter it through their worldview grid and life experiences. Cancer is not like other preventable or more predictable diseases. Because it is so seemingly random and insidious, when faced with cancer, your friends will have to face these questions: What would I do if I had cancer? Will I get it? Will I die this way?

Cancer reminds everyone that life is short and unpredictable and no human being is in control of his or her life. Some people will not be able to visit you because they get slapped in the face with that truth and refuse to confront it. Sadly, some are just repulsed by illness as cancer interrupts their pretty picture of life.

Every person who doesn't come has a reason for staying away. You may be blessed, as I was, to hear some of the reasons why. Others may never reveal their reasons to you. Determined not to grow bitter about the ones who did not come, I asked the Spirit to use my illness to His advantage in their lives. I want to encourage you to adopt that same practice. Only God Himself knows each human heart and the agony it suffers. Every time the absence is felt, use it as an opportunity to pray for freedom from bitterness for yourself and courage for the other person to face the difficulties of life.

God Himself will care for you just as you need. Confess your hurt and loneliness to Him. Grieve the absence of beloved friends. God will walk with you on the journey to a healed and whole heart. He will use those who are available and even those who are unaware of Him to meet your need. At the same time, God will use this experience for the good of your friends and family. Pray for them as their journey is painful, too.

I think the main issue for you, the patient—the one being ignored, unattended, or neglected—is to forgive. In the middle of the biggest battle of your life, you are called to surrender to the emotional pain inflicted by another. The active choice to forgive brings victory over an invader that can rob you of times of enjoyment and freedom. The Bible warns us that this invader can quickly become a root not easily dislodged. Bitterness feels powerful. With caustic remarks or disdainful looks, you can temporarily rise in power over your victimizer. The longer bitterness is lodged in your heart, the more reason you will find to remain bitter. The one who hurt you will never be able to do anything to make up for the pain. Even their request for forgiveness will feel hollow to you as long as you cling to bitterness.

Ask the Lord to give you His grace to forgive. He is able to help you and free you. In the difficulty of forgiveness, you will receive a gift. You will become more aware of how much you are forgiven and how much it cost Jesus to forgive you. You will understand with depth how much you are loved.

BIBLE VERSES TO READ

☐ Hebrews 12:15

☐ Ruth 1:13b; 1:20-21

☐ Genesis 50:15-21

☐ Matthew 18:21-35

☐ James 3:14-18

REFLECTIONS

Bitterness remembers details. Take a minute to reflect on your life and ask the Lord to reveal to you any bitterness you might hold toward someone who has hurt you.

Naomi and Joseph had two different responses to the events of their lives. What made the difference for Joseph? You may need to read starting in Genesis 37.

(Matthew 18:21-35) If we don't forgive, what danger are we in?
(James 3:14-18) What changes in us if we do forgive?

WEEK IN REVIEW

This week's high:

This week's low:

List the names of those who loved you well this week and share a brief description of what they did.

WEEK IN REVIEW

Today I feel . . .

My favorite quote this week is . . .

My favorite Bible verse this week is . . .

JOURNAL PROMPTS

What circumstances are tempting you to be bitter? Has someone turned away from you, have your needs gone unmet, or are you holding on to some hurt? Write a prayer outlining these incidents so that you can see them in black and white.

If forgiveness brings freedom and joy, what makes you resistant to forgive someone who hurt you? Will you choose to lay that resistance aside? Sometimes we must keep going to God for grace and confession until bitterness is gone and we have forgiven.

Often, during our hardest battles, we face an issue that reveals a residual sin that we may miss in the ordinary trials of life. Do not resist looking at this issue. God wants to free you in every way. If you examine your heart and have no bitterness, thank the Lord for giving you freedom. If you do have bitterness, take the time to forgive.

MY PRAYERS THIS WEEK

11

BITTERNESS WEEDING

"Bitterness is like cancer. It eats upon the host."
—Maya Angelou

*W*hile we are on the subject of hurt feelings and broken relationships, and you are in the position to reflect, I think it is a good time to discuss a universal problem of the human heart. It is sneaky, self-righteous, and ever so justifiable. Bitterness is its name.

Bitterness is as insidious as a weed. In fact, the Bible teaches that it can take root in the human heart. It creeps up when you are at your most vulnerable and brings with it an evil sense of power that replaces the helpless hurt of a painful experience.

Let me share a personal experience. Some time ago, I was standing in a group of women, discussing confusion over a change in our circumstances, when bitterness reared its ugly head again. A dear friend repeated some painful episodes that I had with another woman. As if in an out-of-body experience, I heard my own hateful words clothed in self-righteous martyrdom as I joined in and shared more hurtful discussions.

The woman I couldn't get along with is not a heinous unbeliever. She is not an ax murderer or a callous heathen. But I left indelibly printed in the minds of that circle of women a picture of innocent me being attacked viciously by an evil, worthless person. The truth is that she is a capable, valuable woman with years of ministry experience under her belt. She deserves my respect even when I disagree. She is a person made in the image of God, for whom Christ died.

In the flush of vindication, or maybe vengeance is a better word, I forgot the many kind acts of service she did for me. Did I mention some of the pain that she must deal with? No! I just remembered that she didn't hear me, she didn't understand me, and she didn't really like me. I only remembered things that fed my bitterness. When the conversation ended, I heard a little nagging Voice ask, "Have you fully forgiven her? Did that help you deal with your sin?"

Later that week, I shared my shame with Ruth Booth, an older woman in our church who never stopped growing. Gently, she took me to a time in her life of similar struggle. She was mistreated and fell into the temptation to withdraw. The Lord began to speak to her. As Ruth poured out her heart to Him, He revealed the depth of His love to her afresh. The Lord showed her that her desire to be loved was stronger than her desire to love.

During this time, Ruth reflected on the life of the person who was hurting her. She realized how utterly devoid of affection this woman was. Her antagonizer had driven everyone away with her caustic tongue and hurtful manner. Ruth began to release her hold on her bitterness, but she found herself talking about the situation and finding satisfaction in the sympathy and indignation of others. As I had, she relished reliving the hateful moments, surrounded by friends ready to slay the offender. Once again, the Lord smote her heart.

Hadn't He allowed this woman to be brought into her life? Was not He quite capable of removing her? What did Ruth really want? Everyone in her life loved her—except for this one woman. Here was an opportunity to love someone as Jesus did. This was her time to identify with Jesus in His sufferings. Ruth discovered that she mistakenly believed she had a right to bitterness. If she no longer talked about this woman derogatorily, then she could no longer hold onto any control or any sense of logical reason; she would have to let God be her only comfort and her only source of help. Shortly thereafter, just as she began to love this woman and hold her tongue, the woman died. Ruth had few opportunities to love her well. She looked at me sadly and knowingly.

When you get down to it, every one of us must regularly deal with seeds of bitterness. When life hands us blows we cannot explain and did not plan for, we scramble for answers and point accusingly at God. When we are unjustly treated, bitterness has the opportunity to take root as we point at others. We often settle for our fleshly desire for understanding, for advocates, and for being a helpless victim. If we talk long enough and to enough people, someone will water us with sympathy and encourage our outrage. Someone will join in our confusion and point fingers of accusation in the other direction. For a few minutes, we are comforted by the thought of triumphant us and humiliated them. Then that Voice comes, accompanied by a picture of Jesus struggling for breath as He unjustly bore our sins.

Still, we argue. Okay, Lord, we might concede a little to having a bad attitude, but *they* are the real guilty ones. Roseann Coleman once said that we view ourselves more like the Pharisee when we sin, but in fact we are shameless prostitutes. We refuse to see that our wrong response to pain is as obvious in our walk with God as their sin is in their walk with us. How grievous. How fleshly. How natural. The Voice returns, and the picture of Jesus agonizing in pain and emotional torment in separation from God for *my* sin of bitterness flashes again across my mind. Lord, I am undone; I have sinned.

Every one of us must choose to trust God and accept unjust pain and humiliation or we will waste years of energy and resources looking for vindication. Just as Ruth will never know the satisfaction of having loved that woman sufficiently, I will never know how God could have blessed me or others if I had the maturity to release my pain to Him.

Can God really meet us at the point of our greatest humiliation? Can we trust Him to give us grace to manage unexpected, unwanted shifts, to help us rise to the occasion without the shackles of bitterness holding us back? Are we willing to give Him the right to direct our paths, even when that brings with it unjustified pain and confusion? Can you hear bitterness when you relate your pain to others? Can they?

BIBLE VERSES TO READ

☐ Hebrews 12:15

☐ Ruth 1:13b; 1:20-21

☐ Genesis 50:15-21

☐ Matthew 18:21-35

☐ James 3:14-18

REFLECTIONS

Same verses. Same topic. It's that important. Take a few minutes and review your life. Make sure that you have dealt with the hurts of your life properly, forgiving others for hurting you and accepting God's grace to turn the pain into something beautiful. Reread the Hebrews passage and reflect on the ups and down of your life.

Ruth was not in control of her destiny. Neither are we. Has cancer itself made you bitter at this turn in your life? How do you see the goodness of God in this situation?

How might God use your suffering for good, as He did Joseph's? Will you lay it before Him and ask Him to give you insight into not only your healing from bitterness but the effect that it might have on those closest to you? Record your thoughts here. Pray for that outcome.

WEEK IN REVIEW

This week's high:

This week's low:

List the names of those who loved you well this week and share a brief description of what they did.

WEEK IN REVIEW

Today I feel . . .

My favorite quote this week is . . .

My favorite Bible verse this week is . . .

JOURNAL PROMPTS

We can be bitter toward God for allowing us to have cancer. Take a few minutes and honestly examine your heart over this issue. Write out your response here.

The frightful reality that we are not in control of our circumstances can be remedied by surrendering to the One who is in control. Once and for all, lay out before Him whatever is left of your life and invite Him to reveal Himself to you. Read Romans 8 several times and ask for insight as this chapter applies to your current situation. What is one purpose of this trial in your life according to Romans 8?

You have today to live, giving your whole self to God. Will you? Write out your honest prayer to Him. If you are reluctant to give yourself to Him, tell Him. Pour out your heart.

MY PRAYERS THIS WEEK

12

'ONLINESS'

Everything I've ever needed to learn about living dependently
I've learned from a three-year-old.

*E*verything was taken care of. The girls were going to stay with three-year-old Michael while I went to lunch with a friend. They were fixing lunch and planned out their time. As I bent down to kiss Michael goodbye, he began to cry. It wasn't the usual "I'm mad because I want to go, too" bawl. It was a sad, hiccupping sob that came from his heart. Premeditated or not, it stopped me dead in my tracks. With tears streaming down his cheeks, he said, "But Mom, I'll be so 'only' without you."

I drove to lunch knowing exactly how my little boy felt and was touched by that longing need. I hear it in my own heart often. Like a New York taxi driver, as I frantically race from one stop to the next with my involved pre-driving adolescents, I feel my "onliness." Trying to guide the hearts of my children through the torrential flooding of adolescence is akin to a blind woman driving seventy miles per hour on the interstate during rush hour with a busload of roaming two-year-olds! Terrifying does not cover it! Decision-making, juggling schedules, balancing between trusting and protecting, letting go and holding on—parenting pushes me to an awareness of my "onliness." Cancer did that for me, too.

I have never pretended to be a strong, independent woman. Therefore, I have taken it upon myself to learn how to become a better organizer, more efficient house cleaner, and more authoritative parent. In those rare instances when all the ducks line up without even a quack, I've felt my "onliness" swell with all-American pride in great organizational skills. I discovered it is possible to do many things in my own strength. And I've done many! However, the end result echoes like a hollow, empty room. I am lonely in my "onliness."

Cancer stops us in our ever-grasping quest for independence. We are confronted by needs that require us to get help. I remember meeting a Jewish woman at MD Anderson one day, and I heard her recount her upbeat story. It focused on how independent she had been as a single mom with cancer. I grew tired just listening to her. She kept working except on the worst days. Finally, she admitted that she had help from her synagogue. Even in her "onliness," there were people who filled in the gaps.

Don't get me wrong. I am not advocating that we just sit down and demand to be nursed back to health. We are admonished to carry our own load as we reach out to help others carry theirs. Mature adults are capable of carrying their own responsibilities through many seasons of life. Then, as we travel through different experiences, we give a hand to others who need help and encouragement. Biblical independence should lead us to interdependence. Life hands us many opportunities to do that, and it will also hand us opportunities to reach out in need of help. Cancer is that opportunity. As people meet our needs, we are mellowed by gratitude and strengthened through their kindness. In our time of need, God uses people to extend to us tangible evidence of His love. In due time, because of our own awareness of suffering, when we are touched by the needs of others, we are ready and willing to reach into their lives.

I must admit that I could not have been in a better situation during my treatment. Before I even managed to pick up my head through the fog of disbelief, the Lord already began to care for us. What I am about to describe may be much more than you have available to you. I hope that this will give you freedom to speak about your needs and how you could see them being met. If you are part of a church, you may take this chapter to someone and utilize it as a springboard for this type of care through your church to its members as well as those who are needy within the sphere of your influence.

I am a member of a church of about 400 members. My husband and I belong to one of the small groups within the church that meet together for the purposes of applying the teachings of the Bible to our lives and encouraging one another as we practice what we believe. The leader's wife, Diana, and I had been dear friends for several years and shared openly about the issues of our lives.

When we got the diagnosis that my lump was cancerous, Diana was at home with my three-year-old and three homeschooling children. Diana has a unique, God-given gift for making people feel cared for and comforted. She looked at our situation and went to work. When we got the dates for an out-of-state second opinion, she stayed with the children. As we settled into a routine for treatment, she made arrangements for people in our church to drive the children on the days they went to their classes, ensured our oldest had transportation to her public high school, and scheduled childcare for our youngest when I went to the clinic. Diana arranged for meals to be brought to us three times a week during the whole six months! She arrived at our house on a regular basis and did the laundry and mopped the kitchen floor.

When the children were out of line, Diana spoke to them. She stood in the place of my sisters, who all live far away in the Northeast and were unable to come for every situation like that. I threw up only three times in the whole six months of treatment. Diana held my head two of those times. Her role in all of our lives was so tender and practical that it was unanimous among my brothers and sisters that we adopt her! It is because of Diana that I write this chapter.

Another dear friend gave up her summer job so she could take me to my weekly chemo dates. She would drive to Sonic and buy us both a slush, pick me up, and settle us into the chemo room. Eventually, I would fall asleep knowing Brenda was keeping me safe and loved. She was God's comforter to me.

My youngest sister, Laura, finished her school year in Vermont and came to live with us for the first six weeks of my treatment. It felt so good to have someone take care of me who knew how to nurture as my own mother had nurtured. Laura knew when a dropped egg on toast would hit the spot and knew to come in frequently, hand me water, or just chat, straighten the bed, and be normal. She understands my silly sense of humor and would make me laugh. I could feel the children relax as she took the helm and began to calmly and quietly go through the days, following a routine as near as possible to what they were used to doing. I heard quiet conversations mingled with laughter. Laura's curiosity about their lives surprised them and they stopped bickering and listened to each other. She gave Diana a break from the housework and they would swap turns taking me to chemo. She created a deep, loving bond with us that spans the distance of our homes.

Believers are blessed with an objective truth that has nothing to do with ability or luck—it is the promise of the presence of the Holy Spirit to meet any and every circumstance with *all* spiritual blessings from the Heavenlies. God often and most usually uses people to accomplish His purposes. Cancer can be the stage God uses to intermingle His grace through other people in the face of our need. We must not resist in stubborn self-sufficiency. Jesus can transform our self-inflicted, proud, independent perseverance into an opportunity to experience the reality of the Living God during this crisis of cancer.

It is not that hard to humbly seek help and relief in the presence of a loving Father. He is our only hope out of that prison of "onliness."

I was the grateful recipient of much love and forethought. Before I even thought about a need, Diana, Brenda, Laura, and my husband figured out how to meet it. During this time of illness, you will have opportunities to let others help you in ways you could not imagine would ever be necessary. Don't miss the blessing by clinging to your "onliness." Humbly admit what you need and gratefully accept God's gift of love to you through the people in your life.

BIBLE VERSES TO READ

- ☐ 2 Corinthians 1:3-5; comforting us so we may comfort

- ☐ Galatians 6:2-5; carrying one another's burdens

- ☐ 2 Corinthians 9:12-13; supplying the needs of the saints

- ☐ 2 Corinthians 7:6; comforting the humble, comfort by the arrival of Titus

- ☐ 2 Corinthians 4:15-17; grace extended through more and more people increases thanksgiving to God's glory

REFLECTIONS

People who have suffered generally will reach out to sufferers because they are quicker to see the consequences of illness in somebody's life. How have the people around you reached out to you from their own various kinds of suffering?

We are to carry one another's burdens. We cannot do that if we don't know what someone else's burden is. Are you reluctant to share? What are some difficulties you are facing that you could use help with? Logistics of treatment (rides), daily needs (food and cleaning), and help with children or parents are examples of common difficulties.

Paul was comforted by the arrival of Titus during his stay in prison. Who would comfort you if they came? Can you ask them to come?

WEEK IN REVIEW

This week's high:

This week's low:

List the names of those who loved you well this week and share a brief description of what they did.

WEEK IN REVIEW

Today I feel . . .

My favorite quote this week is . . .

My favorite Bible verse this week is . . .

JOURNAL PROMPTS

Have you found it difficult to ask for specific help? Why do you think that it is hard for you to ask for help? If it hasn't been difficult, who did you turn to first for help? Describe that request.

There's a healthy balance between being cared for and being independent. What tasks are you able to do during treatment? What tasks have you delegated to others, or what tasks do you need to delegate to others temporarily?

If people are allowed to give to you, through prayer and tangible help, how will that bring praise and thanksgiving to God?

MY PRAYERS THIS WEEK

13

THE WHOLE PACKAGE

*W*e have a wonderful, loving, chow-retriever named Nick. He greets me every morning with a wag and an expectant move toward the pantry where his dog bones are kept. He gently takes them from me and chomps contentedly while I drink my coffee. When Roger comes in, Nick gets a good-morning fur ruffling. Then we take our respective spots around the room and settle down for some quiet time. One morning, shortly after my cancer diagnosis, the usual ritual performed, we sat trying to avoid eye contact, synchronizing our pain-filled sighs. Nick, in his usual spot beside my chair, slowly stood up and put his golden, lion-like head in my lap and looked at me with warm, sympathetic, brown eyes. Roger and I simultaneously sobbed. Nick became the catalyst for us to begin our journey together into the unknown and unwanted abyss of cancer as our separate tears mingled together over Nick's furry body.

My husband and I met while preparing to go on a study trip around the world. At age thirty, I came to the conclusion that marriage was not going to happen for me. I didn't want to be a bored spinster, so I signed up for a safe adventure. Roger, as a child of missionaries, grew up in Indonesia. He had seen the world several times, and his interest was study.

Through the preparation for this trip, we became good friends. Once, during this period, I called home and told my mom all about Roger and how athletic and competitive he was. I wondered aloud how our differences would work out, as I am more the spectator and cheerleader type. With her classic and serious confidence in me, Mom's words of assurance still make me laugh. "But, Donne, you play croquet!"

Months after the trip, following a particularly intense session in our seminary counseling class, I met Roger's roommate, who noticed my teary demeanor. As soon as he left me, he reported to Rog that I had been crying. Roger's answer shines like a beacon over our life together. He said, "That's just part of the package, Ted, just part of the package!"

Little did Roger know when we took our marriage vows that the part of the package labeled "in sickness and in health" would mean facing cancer. But not once has he wavered in his love and acceptance of me. In fact, his loving commitment was best illustrated on a date we had in Italy.

We were missionaries with three small children. In the midst of language study, toddler chaos, and the enormous task of living in a foreign culture, we had little time for us, so Roger planned a whole day of skiing by ourselves in the Italian Alps. This Maine girl had only downhill skied twice, both times on the gentle slopes of North Carolina. I loved everything about skiing and was naively confident about the prospects of such a glorious adventure.

We took the box lift up the hill with about twenty others. Roger found the practice slope for me, and after I had done it a few times, he called me to come down the hill. Looking at it from the top, the slope seemed to be a ninety-degree angle with a sheer drop to the left. There was a thin glaze of ice shimmering on the top. The only thing melting was my confidence. I said to Roger, "I cannot do this. Where's the easy slope?"

Into the whiteness, Roger said, "Donne, this is the easy slope. There is no other way down. Come on, you can do this." I looked at him and I looked at the slope. Skiers were beginning to whiz by me, looking a bit irritated with my in-the-middle-of-the-path position. I took a tentative lean, and all too soon, the ground was moving much too fast for me. I promptly sat down to avoid the crashing death I knew was inevitably waiting.

Now Roger began to look a bit irritated with my in-the-middle-of-the-path position as skiers were agilely maneuvering around me at an alarmingly fast rate. I stood up and decided to try again. Another six feet and the ground again began moving too fast for me, so I did the only thing I knew that brought a semblance of control; I sat down. "I am stuck. I cannot do this."

No amount of cajoling touched my fear-motivated decision. Finally, my athletic husband, who never met a sport he could not conquer, crossed the path to me, silently and laboriously turned his skis in a downhill direction, and placed them in a *V* in front. Over his shoulder, he said, "Donne, put your skis inside mine. Then, put your arms around my waist. I will carry you down as slowly as possible." As if in a dream, I complied. My relief was palpable.

It was a beautiful, cold, clear day. The snow sparkled in the sun. Other people whizzed past us at the speed of light. They missed the snow sifting through the boughs of the fir trees. They didn't see the birds amid the greenery. I was safely and securely escorted by my daredevil husband to the bottom without reproach or shame. He took me, my fear, and my inability to ski safely to the parking lot. This same man, twelve years later, did the same thing for me down the frightening slope named cancer.

Rog became my brain. He read, researched, and filtered through options and treatments. He gave me the bottom line of each one and his opinion of what was best. Arm in arm, we walked the path before us. When I was particularly fearful, he reminded me that we were doing the best known treatment and would not budge in his conviction that I should hold to it. He held me through tears and throwing up. He asked questions and made suggestions, all the while feeling the weight of my life leaning into his, knowing I was longing to be whole and beside him rather than needing to be carried. It became part of the package he chose when we married.

You may not have someone like Roger in your life who will give you that kind of support, but I do know that Jesus can meet your needs in as tangible a way as He used Roger to meet mine. As you lean into this unknown abyss, close your eyes and picture yourself leaning into the back of someone who lovingly holds your life in His hands and will carry you safely down this slope to the end. He will take on your whole package!

BIBLE VERSES TO READ

☐ Ephesians 1:3-5

☐ Psalm 139:1-6

☐ Psalm 139:7-12

☐ Psalm 139:13-16

☐ 1 Peter 2:9-10

REFLECTIONS

Looking at Ephesians 1:3-5, when did the Lord first think about you? How precious are you to the Lord of the Universe?

(Psalm 139:1-6) How much of your "whole package" was the Lord aware of when He made you? Can you trust that He knew you would suffer with cancer and longed to turn it into good for you and a chance for you to know Him better?

(1 Peter 2:9-10) Chemo and the struggle with cancer can run amuck with your emotions. Can you record instances of hope and light that you have experienced as God has led you through this trial?

WEEK IN REVIEW

This week's high:

This week's low:

List the names of those who loved you well this week and share a brief description of what they did.

WEEK IN REVIEW

Today I feel . . .

My favorite quote this week is . . .

My favorite Bible verse this week is . . .

JOURNAL PROMPTS

If you could sit down face to face with the Lord, what would you like to ask Him about cancer in your life?

Reflect back over your life. List ways that God has rescued you from other situations or led you through them to get you to a better place.

What are the components of your life that make up your whole package and make it hard for you to believe that you are truly loved?

MY PRAYERS THIS WEEK

14

TAKING CARE OF YOUR CAREGIVERS

"Edisto created the Snowberger family motto, 'We live to serve.'"
—Each Little Bird That Sings

*M*y mother is the ultimate caregiver. For all her married life, she has had the responsibility of caring for aging parents, in-laws, and various and sundry relatives while simultaneously managing a family of six children. Throughout her responsibilities, she maintained her gentle spirit and loving care. As a child, I found excuses to stay home from school, and she would bring me tea and toast, fix my bed, and chat for a minute. She knew how to give that "Relax, you are loved, you are healing" sensation. When I was a teen, she understood that sometimes, I just needed to stay home, stop the rat race long enough to get a plan, and start over again.

When Grampy rolled a 500-pound lawnmower over onto himself, she was watching and moved it to rescue him. Then she cared for his every need until he was once again mobile and getting himself into more scrapes! When her mother joined our household, Mom was glad for the help. All the while, she washed Nana's hair and rolled it. She rubbed her back. She made the adjustments you need to make to allow for another person to be in your home. Then, twenty years later, as Nana was dying, Mom sat by Nana's bed and helped her do it with dignity. She loved with grace and without resentment. Since that time, two of her sisters died. Another has been weak and needing help. Who was there for them? My mom. After hospital stays, they came to her. She cared for them. She says it's what you're supposed to do. I say it is heroic.

More than once as a young mother, feeling particularly harried from my own chaos, I asked Mom how she kept it up. She said, "Your dad always made sure to take me out." Therein lies a great secret of endurance. Someone paid attention to the needs of the caregiver. That is what this chapter is all about. Unless you are totally isolated, someone in your life is helping you out during this time. Most of us have many people. From the chemotherapy nurse to your spouse, caregivers provide a wide range of services to help us through this illness. Without them, our treatment would be much more difficult.

Take a minute right now and make a mental list of the different people who touched your life today in some sort of service to you. Wonder what went through their minds and hearts as they reached out. Each one of them has busy lives of their own—with needs and hurts and dreams—but they placed themselves in your life for your good. Some of them do it for a living. Many do it because they love you. Even when you are ill, you can give back to them in many ways.

All of the nurses who treated me during chemotherapy were professional, highly trained, and personable. They were not overly sympathetic, nor were they cold and indifferent. I saw them hold each other and cry when they received news of a patient's death. I watched the banter and could figure out who was irritating whom as, week after week, they dealt with a flood of ill people. During emergencies, they became one, seemingly reading each other's minds. They each had "their" patients. They knew which one of them could and would handle the cantankerous, the wobbly veins, the demanding. Each of my nurses had different stories. One was single. Three had young families. All of them loved a good laugh and chocolate! Have you thought about your nurses this week? How are they doing?

Acknowledging the sacrifices that an individual has made to be there for you is a good place to start caring for your caregiver. Be conscious of the amount of time your care is demanding. No one has to be there for you. No one person needs to be consumed and totally immersed in you! Treat them accordingly. Each of your caregivers, even your spouse, has a life and needs. From taking care of household bills and cleaning to taking a walk and a long bubble bath, your helper needs time for rejuvenation and refreshment. Roger found release from the stress by riding a bicycle. Diana maintained her swim class at the YMCA.

Merely putting yourself in their shoes and being grateful connects to the heart of the giver like nothing else. It is not a difficult exercise. Remember to appreciate your caregivers by saying a simple thank-you for their time, their thoughtfulness, and their interest in you. We have all heard stories of spouses who are abandoned during illness and of children who walk away in the time of their parent's need. There are still others who *are* helping. They will be encouraged by your appreciation. As best you can, urge your caregivers to take care of themselves and keep up with their own activities. Send them out to do that.

It is normal for resentment to flare up when someone is ill and needy. You are that someone. Don't be taken by surprise or wounded by it. The difficulty of the circumstances is the real culprit. Assuring your caregiver of your appreciation and doing all you can to ensure they are getting support from others and taking care of themselves will place the focus on the circumstance and not on your relationship. As best as you can, be aware of how much time any one individual is giving to you. Urge them to do something else at regular intervals. It may prevent resentment from rearing its ugly head.

BIBLE VERSES TO READ

☐ Colossians 3:15

☐ 2 Corinthians 4:15-16

☐ Colossians 4:2

REFLECTIONS

When your life is in chaos, how do you allow the peace of Christ to rule? How can you accept your calling? List what and who you have to be thankful for below.

(2 Corinthians 4:15) How is grace reaching others through your situation? Is it? How can you extend grace to your caregivers?

(Colossians 4:2) Devoting oneself to prayer takes time and energy. Do you have it? Pray for your caregivers and watch how your love for them grows.

WEEK IN REVIEW

This week's high:

This week's low:

List the names of those who loved you well this week and share a brief description of what they did.

WEEK IN REVIEW

Today I feel . . .

My favorite quote this week is . . .

My favorite Bible verse this week is . . .

JOURNAL PROMPTS

Sometimes it's difficult to be grateful. Work hard at it this week. Note especially the things your caregivers do to help that you didn't ask them to do.

How have you encouraged your caregiver to take a break from your constant needs?

It's tempting to sulk in anger at this situation. It's tempting to lash out at the ones closest to you when they don't seem to realize what this situation is costing you. Have you done either one of those things? How can you repair the damage you may have done in your relationships with the ones who are caring for you?

MY PRAYERS THIS WEEK

15

ENDURANCE THROUGH THE VALLEY OF THE SHADOW OF DEATH

*W*hat a name for the last chapter of a book about the unexpected trials of cancer! What must you endure? How can you endure if your life is hanging in the balance? The challenge, as in all trials, is to hold onto our faith in the midst of all circumstances. It is trusting that the Lord is holding onto us when we must endure illness and suffering. When our lives have been put on hold and completely rearranged, our faith must endure.

Psalm 23 says, "Yea, though I walk through the valley of the shadow of death, I will fear no evil, for Thou art with me." Say this out loud and loudly when you are being assaulted with fear and what-ifs. Practice verbalizing that you trust in the One who has loved you since before the world began. Bring your thoughts captive to the truths that you are loved, God is with you, and He will help your faith endure until He calls you home.

As I started the book with the brevity of life, I want to remind you at the end of the book that we are not promised long lives. What we are promised is the presence of the Living God throughout our trials to help us, guide us, and meet the needs of our souls. While our chemo-filled bodies may not feel His presence, the Bible assures us that He is hovering over us with care. Nothing can separate us from the love of God in Christ Jesus.

Romans 8:38-39 says, "For I am persuaded that not even death or life, angels or rulers, things present or things to come, hostile powers, height or depth, or any other created thing will have the power to separate us from the love of God that is Christ Jesus our Lord!" He perfects us and chooses to grow our trust in Him through these trials in a daily relationship with Him. What must endure is our open heart to Him, our trust in His Word, and our willingness to lay our lives in His hands to bring glory to Him. That is the biggest challenge of cancer.

No one is going to live in their bodies forever. We each must let go of this earthly, decaying shell in order to receive the new body and new life planned for us before the world began. Just as the end of a pregnancy is filled with the dread of birth, the pregnant woman also is looking forward to holding new life in her arms and all the breathtaking love that goes with it. One purpose of our suffering is to help us to see beyond the earthly bond our bodies have in this life to the new life promised us in the future. We have a future, and it will be better than the one we imagined before cancer struck. It will be better than anything we could ask for. Read about it. Think hard about it. As you heal from this episode in your life, you will bear in your body the reminders that your life here on earth is temporary. That's not a bad thing. Keep your mind on heaven, and your priorities will reflect the good changes necessary to live a meaningful life.

Cancer is hard. Don't let me make you think I don't get it. There are tears, grieving, anger, anguish, and fear. So much fear. After all of the emotions have run their course, I pray your faith will blossom and endure, my friend. The One who loves you most is hovering over you with great care. Ask Him to show you the way, to give you His peace, to open doors of help and healing, and to keep your focus on Him and the future. May the God of peace reign supreme in your heart as you endure these light afflictions until we meet Him face to face.

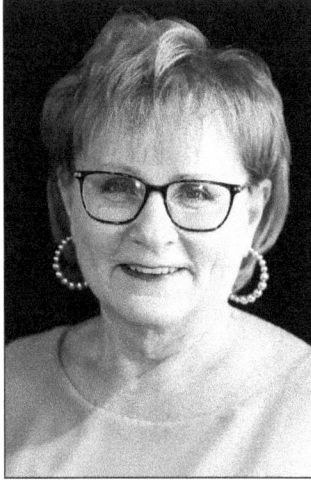

ABOUT THE AUTHOR

A native of Maine, Donne Smith graduated from Columbia Bible College/Columbia International University with a BA in Bible teaching and a master's in Christian education. She taught Bible in a public school in North Carolina for four years. While pursuing her master's degree, she met her husband, Roger. They spent six years on a church-planting team in Italy with TEAM.

Donne is the mother of four children and the grandmother of seven (so far). She and her husband live in Jackson, Tennessee, and travel to Maine every summer to visit her family there.

www.ingramcontent.com/pod-product-compliance
Lightning Source LLC
Chambersburg PA
CBHW042346030426
42335CB00031B/3475